Pinky Promise

A Daily Dose of Faith,

Hope and Inspiration

DISCLAIMER

Although you may find the stories and advice useful, the book is sold with the understanding that neither the authors nor the Women Wellness Lounge are engaged in presenting any legal, relationship, financial, emotional, or health advice. The purpose of this book is to educate and entertain. The authors and publishers shall neither assume liability nor responsibility for anyone with respect to any loss or damage caused directly or indirectly by the information in the book.

Any person who is experiencing financial, anxiety, depression, health, mental health, or relationship issues should consult with a licensed therapist, advisor, licensed psychologist, or other qualified professional before commencing into anything described in this book.

Table of Contents

Pinky Promise

Foreword

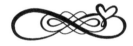

In the face of adversity, courage blossoms. This book is a beacon of hope for the remarkable women navigating the challenging terrain of breast cancer. As you embark on this resilience journey, may these pages illuminate the strength within, fostering inspiration and unwavering optimism. Together, let us celebrate the indomitable spirit that binds us all and the transformative power of hope in the face of uncertainty.

Visionary Author,
Delayna Watkins
Founder, Women's Wellness Lounge
www.womenswellnesslounge.org
In strength and remembrance
Penny Judkins
Celestine Harris
Tara Pannell
Vanessa Davis

Cancer Can Be a Blessing

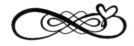

My pink sisters, hearing the words, **"You have breast cancer,"** can be very devastating. Once you have absorbed those words, which may take a while, feel free to cry, scream, or do whatever you need to overcome the shock. I know this may sound crazy, but as you travel through this journey, I want you to look at some of the positive things that have been happening in your life since being diagnosed. I suggest you keep a journal to see how far you have come and what positive changes have happened to you personally and to others.

As you travel through your breast cancer journey, you will find out that cancer could very well end up being a blessing instead of a curse. Cancer will teach you many valuable lessons you may not have otherwise received. Cancer will teach you many things, not just about yourself but also about other people in your life. Cancer can show you how much you are loved. When you are independent, I know reaching out to others who want to assist you during this challenging time is difficult. However, please know you will bring joy and happiness to those who want to assist you through your journey. Not only will you hear and see the joy in their voice and their face, but you will also see the bright, beautiful smiles you put on their face because you have allowed them to do something that was so important to them...SERVING YOU!

Cancer will teach you to say no without guilt and not waste energy on toxic people because you are number ONE!

Sisters, welcome to an awesome community....one that you don't want to volunteer to join but one that is powerful and full of love and support.

Once your cancer journey is over, assist other women through their journey so you can give them hope, encouragement, and inspiration.

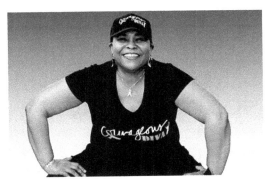

Barbara Palmer

Two-Time 20-year Breast Cancer Survivor,
Author, Patient Advocate

2003 and 2013

Embracing the Journey: Finding Light & Strength in the Face of Breast Cancer

Those Four Words

I was on the phone with my doctor. They usually didn't do this, but she'd let me call in because I'd already spent so much money on copays and other fees for testing and screenings I couldn't afford to go back into the office. One of my sister-friends, Delayna Watkins, a nurse, was on the telehealth call with us. The doctor said the words no one ever wants to hear. You have breast cancer. She tried her best to help me understand what I was facing, but I couldn't digest everything. I remember her saying highly aggressive, late stage 3, rare, rapid spreading, inflammatory, triple-negative breast cancer. My sister-friend helped me process the diagnosis after the doctor hung up. In one phone call, my life changed so drastically. I needed help.

I remember the moment. I remember the feeling. Fear engulfed my spirit. I wish I could say that I was strong and faith-filled when I heard those words, but I can't, and I wasn't. I felt emotionally paralyzed. I had so many thoughts racing through my mind. I was traumatized. I was angry. Of course, I was familiar with the disease and even knew people who had it, but I didn't understand it in relation to me and my life. I was so hurt and confused. What did this mean for me? Would I die at an early age like my mother? What would happen to my children? They were dependent on me. Would I be able to work to support them? How would I pay my bills? Was this curable? How do I tell them? How will they take it? How do I wake up from this nightmare? What if I don't wake up tomorrow morning?

I felt so alone like no one understood what I was going through. That's why I want you to know that you are not alone. I know what it's like to be shaken to your core and feel like you've lost control of your life. It can be overwhelming. But amidst the fear, the uncertainty, and the challenges that lie ahead or that you are dealing with right now, please know that there is light and hope.

Facing the Physical Challenges

Courage and persistence were needed from the onset of the journey. This call with the doctor was the culmination of two months of testing, false diagnoses, uncertainty, and advocating for the proper tests to be performed. The lump had grown to 12 centimeters, and it appeared like a cyst on one side and a hardened tumor on the other. My breast skin turned an angry-looking red-orange color, and it was extremely heavy. It looked like a third breast. I was happy to finally learn what was wrong with me so I could get help, but I was heartbroken because of what was wrong with me.

I made it in to see my oncologist and learned more about my diagnosis. I learned that inflammatory breast cancer is very rare. In my research, I found that it only made up for one to five percent of breast cancer cases in the U.S. It is difficult to detect, and once detected, it is usually in late stage 3 because the cancer cells have already grown into the skin. Inflammatory coupled with triple-negative breast cancer made this significantly more aggressive.

This was hard for me to hear. She had to write everything out for me. My brain would not process anything; she spoke a language I didn't understand. Of all the information she provided, what stood out the most was that I would have to get my breast removed, and my hair would fall out by my second chemo visit. The treatment included three chemo drugs, and one of them was called 'the red devil.'

Now, the medicine I took was Tylenol now and then. Everything else was curable with juice and vegetables. This level of drugs was unreal.

I was proactive and did things to empower myself before the first chemo treatment. I nurtured and strengthened my immune system; I got my hair cut low so the hair loss wouldn't be a traumatic shock, and I launched my first book before my first treatment. I am happy I took those steps because the first treatment wiped me out. I'd never felt so low in energy and weak.

To my surprise, when I went for my first chemo session, there were so many people there. The visit was long. I sat for over four hours, having the drugs administered. There were the pre-drugs to prep my system and then the big dogs. There was a lot of time to think in that session and others. I am so grateful that someone was always with me. The other patients and their loved ones were usually friendly. I would read, watch TV, or fall asleep because I was so weak and many times ill. I learned that everyone had different physical experiences and different types of treatment and received their treatment at different frequencies.

Radiation was less taxing on my body, but the aftereffects were exhausting. The surgeries were the most physically, mentally, and emotionally complex experiences I'd ever endured. In five years, I underwent 9 surgeries related to my diagnosis. I experienced the physical metamorphosis of my body but also got to witness its God-given strength and ability to heal.

This led me to increase my resilience, perseverance, self-esteem, self-love, and confidence.

Battling the Inner Shadows: The Mental and Emotional Journey

I shared with someone that my cancer journey was devastating. She told me I should re-language my experience because other people going through it would hold on to my words. It may disempower them. That didn't feel right to me.

Although challenging, I want to be authentic and vulnerable and share my truth. I didn't want to hide the uncomfortable or the ugly because you may experience it. And I need you to know that it is part of the journey. You don't have to hide. If you ignore it, you will further stress your immune system and won't reach out for the support you need. We strive to learn lessons, be strong, upbeat, faith-filled, strong, laugh, and have fun. If you are like me, it took some work to get to that space. I must be honest here; the physical changes took me down a depressing mental and emotional path. And I sought help.

I had to have both breasts removed and a partial hysterectomy because of my BRACA gene. Psychotherapy helped me understand, work through how I was responding, and provide methods of coping and healing. While I understood that the surgeries would help save my life, it didn't relieve the grief I felt.

My breast had a deep meaning for me that I needed to acknowledge. I breastfed all four children; it was a special connection and bond. I felt the love and milk flowing from my body into theirs. I watched them develop and grow from the nurturance that I provided. My breasts were also a sensual and sexual part of me. I don't have nipples, nor do I have feelings in my reconstructed breasts.

The wildly sensual sensations I once experienced through my breasts, are no more. I undoubtedly felt a sense of loss and grief, and I felt less attractive. Therapy helped me to find other ways to connect with my sense of womanhood and beauty and build my self-esteem and confidence. The emotional journey was a rollercoaster ride. Please know that it is okay to feel a range of emotions: fear, anxiety, grief, gratefulness, happiness, and joy. It is okay to be vulnerable. Feeling afraid and acknowledging that the journey was tough was okay. However, don't be consumed by fear.

Light on the Journey

Amidst the challenges of a diagnosis, treatments, procedures, loss of control in your life, and multiple changes, there is also light on the path. While this journey can be daunting, it can bring unexpected gifts and blessings.

For me, one of the most beautiful aspects of this journey was the incredible community of support. I was surrounded by people who offered unwavering love, encouragement, and support for me and my children. I also made new connections and friendships. In those moments, I realized that we are never truly alone.

This journey also gave me the opportunity for self-discovery and personal growth. Facing a breast cancer diagnosis requires a level of strength and courage that you may not have known you possessed. You will find newfound passions, talents, purpose, resilience, perseverance, and determination as you navigate treatments and procedures. You will also find a deeper appreciation for the small moments in life and a renewed sense of purpose and gratitude.

Lastly, remember the importance of celebrating victories, no matter how small. Celebrate the moments you can stand up straight, walk to the bathroom, walk through the supermarket, hold down a portion of your meal, or when your first hair grows back. Celebrate! Whether completing a round of treatment or reaching out to others for support, every step forward counts.

As you turn the page to the next chapter, may you find continued strength, hope, beauty, and resilience. Remember that you are enough, just as you are, everything you need is within you, and that your journey is uniquely yours. Embrace it with open arms, and let your light shine bright.

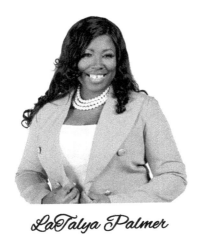

LaTalya Palmer

Breast Cancer Survivor, Author, Coach

The Day of Change

On July 26, 2021, my life changed forever....

Thisis the day I was diagnosed with breast cancer. It was an ordinary day like no other. I worked in the emergency department on a 12-hour shift, caring for patients. I have been a board-certified emergency medicine physician assistant in clinical practice since 2012. I received the devastating news of a cancer diagnosis by an email alert. I had been expecting a phone call from a physician about my biopsy results, as told by the radiologist a couple of days beforehand.

I had felt a lump in my left breast about a month prior. I didn't think of any significance after discovering the lump. Not long ago, I stopped breastfeeding my one-year-old baby girl. I always knew and assumed, like most other women, that breastfeeding would create lumpy breasts. I just figured it was a residual breastfeeding milk cyst. A couple more weeks passed by, and I still felt a lump and asked my husband to palpate the area as well. He agreed that I should get it checked out. About a week later, I set up a virtual appointment and was able to have a mammogram and sonogram scheduled within a couple of weeks. The lump was mildly painful but firm. I was always taught during medical training that breast cancer lumps are usually painless. As a result, the mild pain sensation I felt when the lump was touched added to my feelings of thinking this breast lump was benign. Leading up to the mammogram appointment, I was somewhat nervous. I was 36 years old and didn't expect to have a mammogram for another four years at a minimum. The experience of having my first mammogram was not the most pleasant feeling. Before the mammogram started, the technician verified my age several times and asked the radiologist if I still needed the mammogram. She returned to the room and said, "The radiologist doesn't feel you need to have the mammogram yet because of your age, and I see here that you recently stopped breastfeeding. We should do the sonogram." I replied "NO" and wanted to proceed with the mammogram as ordered. I did experience some discomfort, but nothing intolerable. My nerves were the most pressing ailment of the visit. I did see the breast lesion on the screen, but again, I was only thinking..." This is just a milk cyst." About two days later, I received the mammogram report findings stating, "Benign appearing galactocele consistent with patient's reported history of recent breastfeeding. Repeat sonogram in three months." I was reassured after reading this report. I went on with my everyday life activities. In another two days, another radiologist called me to say, "After reviewing the images on a double look, the margins on this mass look suspicious, and you should have a biopsy." My heart sank! I immediately knew there was a chance of me now having breast cancer and that this was not a simple benign galactocele (milk cyst). I was frantic and impatient at that point. I was upset, mad, and crying! I couldn't wait to be contacted by the breast care specialist as instructed by the overreading radiologist. I dialed into the breast center right away to schedule a biopsy. My husband drove me to the breast biopsy appointment because I needed moral support.

Unfortunately, my husband could not stay with me during the procedure due to COVID-19 visitor restrictions. As a result, I had endured the unsteadiness of the feelings associated with this biopsy alone! I began to pray as I was lying on the procedure table. The radiologist was pleasant and talked to me a great deal. As he started the sonogram before the biopsy, I was also looking at the screen and remember saying to him, "Those margins do look irregular and suspicious."

We also started a conversation about my profession as a medical provider, so now he talked to me in more depth about the procedure. I was still hopeful at that point and thinking, "Ok, he will try to aspirate this cyst first, and if milk is drained, then we know it's not cancerous and can stop the procedure." Well unfortunately, the physician was not able to aspirate any fluid from the breast lesion, and he proceeded to do the complete biopsy. I immediately began to cry because it was not a benign finding. The radiologist tried his best to reassure me and stated, "Let's still wait for pathology because this can be another type of benign cyst. You will get a phone call to discuss the results in about three days." The biopsy was done on a Friday, and I just remembered having a very long and dreary weekend.

Three days later, on July 26, 2021, about four hours into my 12-hour shift, about 3:40 in the afternoon, I received the dreaded news very insensitively. I RECEIVED MY BREAST CANCER DIAGNOSIS FROM A PHONE ALERT PATIENT PORTAL EMAIL NOTIFICATION! I was in the middle of draining a breast abscess from one of my patients! I just logged in quickly, thinking this was probably another type of alert. I had no idea I would be checking results on my phone that would forever change my life. I looked at the report and read the pathology findings showing triple-negative breast cancer, grade 3. My heart dropped! I dropped everything and went to the physician's lounge to pull up the report on a desktop because I was thinking, "This has to be a mistake, or I am not reading this clearly." I printed out the report and read it multiple times and could not believe it! I asked my attending supervising physician working with me that day to review my report to ensure this was correct. I barely knew my attending physician then because I had recently started working at this new hospital a few weeks prior. He read it as well and confirmed the horrific news. I grabbed my phone again and tried to dial Kaiser Permanente Breast Center, but I could not reach a physician directly. I could not even think clearly at that point and was erratic! I left work and went home. I am unsure how I made it home because it was all blurry. Thankfully, I only lived 15 min away from the hospital.

I sat in the car for a while when I pulled into the driveway. I paged the physician and was speaking to an on-call nurse. She confirmed the results, but I demanded to speak to a physician to confirm such devastating news. My husband exited the driveway and immediately dropped to the ground in tears. He knew something was wrong because I was home 8 hours early from work, which had never happened. I never spoke to a physician that day. I told the nurse that the radiologist said someone would call me with the results. I wasn't supposed to receive an email notification. She then told me that sometimes patients receive results electronically before the physician reviews them because of a recent law passage. The CURES Act passed in

2021, requires all hospitals and physicians to make test results available to patients via online portals as soon as they are published. As an ER provider, I knew that my clinical notes were made available to patients online as soon I signed the chart, but I had no idea that this was the impact. I was receiving a cancer diagnosis from a portal notification without the proper confirmation from a physician and with counseling regrading such a sensitive and scary diagnosis. At that moment, I realized I was no longer just a Physician Assistant; I was now a patient, too.

I received a phone call from a radiologist the following day at 8 am confirming the diagnosis. He was very cut and dry. He had no emotion tied into the short conversation and just told me the breast cancer nurse navigator would contact me. I was emotionally torn over the next few days and was in a deep, somber mood. About a week later, I had a multi-disciplinary appointment with the medical team about the next steps. I don't remember recalling much information during that visit. My husband was more of my eyes and ears because I was still in shock and didn't retain much information. As some time progressed, as I went through more testing and, most importantly, the staging PET scan, I grew weaker mentally, spiritually, and emotionally. My PET scan results showed that I was stage 3c. My tumor was 5.5 cm and had spread into multiple lymph nodes in my axilla and neck region.

The only saving grace was no metastasis into my organs. I went back to work as I waited for my chemo start date and even resumed work just two days after my port placement. I wanted to keep myself mentally distracted by doing what I love: caring for patients. I worked until two days before chemotherapy initiation treatments. I remember the last shift I worked before chemo; there was an African American woman in her 60s that I was evaluating in the ER. She presented with complaints of back pain and had a history of breast cancer "in remission." I ordered a CT scan, and my heart dropped when the CT report read that she had metastatic bony lesions in her spine. I couldn't handle it! I burst into tears and ran out of the emergency department. I had to tell the attending physician I was working with that day to take over that patient, and again, I needed to go home. I felt like a complete failure and empty inside. I could not face that sweet patient of mine and tell her the cancer had come back and was metastatic. I couldn't face her with the same condition that I had in the midst of a new scary diagnosis like herself. Beforehand, I have evaluated dozens of patients with cancer histories and have even diagnosed new incidental cancer conditions by remaining a diligent provider. Of course, I never liked to be the bearer of bad news but having cancer myself now ultimately affected me differently. I was more sensitive to the condition now and felt a sense of heightened connection that I never felt before. I was more understanding and empathetic. It felt very similar to when I became a parent for the first time seven years ago. I would always say to myself, "Gosh, some of these parents are overreacting when their children are brought into the ER for minor injuries or illnesses." However, I clearly understood why parents felt the way they did and reacted in that manner when I became a parent, too. It clicked, and becoming a parent made me a better clinician with more understanding. I take that same experience with me now as I am still battling for my life as a Stage 3C Triple Negative Breast Cancer Patient.

It took me a long time to process that I was a cancer patient. How could this be? I am a licensed healthcare professional. I am the person who takes care of patients; how did the roles flip? That was the most significant part of it all for me to digest. I felt vulnerable and weak. After about 8weeks of chemo, an epiphany came to me. I felt helpless but wanted to do something to help patients during my cancer treatment journey. The healthcare provider was still alive within me, and I needed to do something to make me feel fulfilled somehow. I decided to start posting videos about my diagnosis in hopes that it would reach another woman who looks like me and is the same age. I felt people needed to know not to wait until their 40th birthday for a mammogram. Get a mammogram now! Early detection saves lives.

No one pushed this health recommendation to me, and even through my PA college education, I was always taught mammograms don't start until age 40. Well, the recommendations and those schoolbooks were wrong. Here I am at the age of 36, without any known family history of breast cancer, with a new diagnosis of the most aggressive form of breast cancer. It wasn't until after I was diagnosed and started posting videos on social media that I found out that I did have a paternal family history of breast cancer. I always knew my paternal grandmother died of some form of gynecological cancer, but it wasn't breast cancer. She never really discussed her health history, as many African American families do not reveal health conditions. I discovered there's a solid paternal linkage of various cancers, including the pancreas, breast, and cervical. It was still unclear after speaking with some family members about which family member had what condition because it was assumed to be "quiet about people's business." I decided this narrative had to change beginning with me. After growing a stronger social media presence, I started receiving feedback from random women asking me for more advice, sharing their stories, and providing positive feedback. Since I couldn't serve patients directly in the ED while I was on leave from work receiving chemo, I figured I could reach more via social media. I have become stronger with advocacy work and breast cancer awareness efforts. I was introduced to Tigerlily Foundation via email by a friend of Maimah's and quickly found myself in the angel advocate program.

I started my organization to help foster my breast cancer awareness efforts with online speaking panels, community events, TV campaigns, etc. I felt like God was using me for a reason, and I became more positive about my journey and diagnosis. I have completed 16 weeks of chemo and 25 sessions of radiation like a champ. I went through a bilateral mastectomy three months ago and had another 6-8 months left of oral chemotherapy. My mastectomy went well, and it showed that all 26 of my lymph nodes removed were cancer-free! They were able to remove the tumor surgically with the breast tissue, and now I must complete oral chemo for any circulating and/or microscopic residual cancer cells in my bloodstream. I am not happy about the upcoming remainder of treatments, but I am hopeful that it will continue to work as my other treatments have. My tumor decreased in size from 5.5 cm down to 1.6 cm at the time of surgery. I am very grateful and blessed for that response from chemo because it signified that it worked in my body to fight cancer cells. I am hopeful, grateful, blessed, humble, and positive that I will be declared cancer-free forever to be here for my three daughters to flourish in life. I still have a lot to live for, and I travel the world with my loving husband, best friend, and biggest supporter. I would not be able to get through this at all without him! Cancer is not just a physical diagnosis. It also affects your mental, emotional, spiritual, and financial state. It also affects your loved ones, and as a cancer thriver, you need a support system and mental health treatment, too. I have good and bad days but thrive and will not stop until the wheels fall off! I have dedicated myself to helping to eradicate breast cancer and mainly decrease the higher mortality associated with Black Breast Cancer. I owe this to my three daughters, whom I pray will never have to experience what I am going through in this life journey.

To all my breasties worldwide, don't forget to fight and count your blessings because you are blessed, my lovelies. Lose yourself in helping others feel better, and always remember to be kind to yourselves.

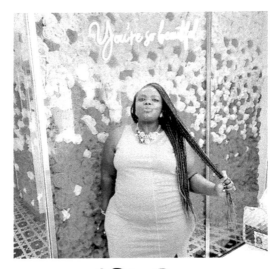

LaToya Bolds

Breast Cancer Survivor, Patient Advocate

"Love Me Some Me"

Psalm 118:17-20

"I didn't die. I lived. And now I'm telling the world what GOD did. GOD tested me; he pushed me hard, but he didn't hand me over to Death." The Message Bible

1. Create a theme, quote, etc., for yourself.
   Remember, your diagnosis is not a death sentence, but it's a license to live.

2. Your living environment should be a place of peace, neat and clean. I love flowers. I change my dining room and kitchen table according to the season. Tip: The Dollar Store has wonderful table settings.

3. Choose at least one day per week to avoid watching and listening to negative news, shows, etc. Sunday is my Sabbath when I attend church, read, color, or watch a good movie.

4. Join a breast cancer support group. This is a safe place where you can discuss with other survivors.

5. Create a team. Do not try to take this journey alone. If possible, have at least two breast cancer survivors on your team. You need people who are confidential and will provide encouragement for you. You don't need people to feel sorry for you.

6. Write your story. Purchase a beautiful journal and write your thoughts, which you can later turn into a book.

7. Change your eating habits by eating more plant-based foods. Keep a food journal: record the date, time you eat, what you eat, weight/BMI, and how much water you drink daily.

8. Avoid negative people. Go where you are celebrated and not tolerated.

In the words of Jill Scott, "I'm living my life like it's golden."

Enjoy your journey!!

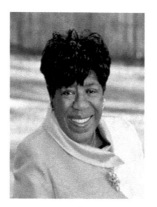

Ruth Travis

16-year breast cancer survivor

Diagnosed November 27, 2007: Zero stage with 100% survival. I was diagnosed two days before my 62nd birthday. I hadn't had a mammogram since age 40.

Greater Is Within Me

When I was first diagnosed with breast cancer, the first thing I remembered was that people would call it the "Big C," as if there was no hope. But I remembered looking up to God, saying, "The only Big

C I know, God, is Jesus Christ. For greater is He that is in me than he that is in the world."

I encourage you to pull strength from knowing that God is greater than anything you will ever face, even cancer. It is not of our strength that we can endure life's challenges, but the "Greater that is within me" enables us to stand, endure, keep moving, and continue to live.

During our journey, we don't have to worry about being strong. Don't add that level of stress to yourself. The only strength we need is to believe that God has us in the palm of His hands, knows our end from the beginning, and is a good Father.

Cancer cannot defeat me because Greater is within me.

Chemotherapy cannot take my strength because Greater is within me.

Radiation is not enough to stop me because Greater is within me.

Because of the Greater within me, I am assured that I WIN!

Whether I WIN on this side or I WIN on the other side, I WIN!

Because Greater is within me!

1 John 4:4

"Ye are of God, little children, and have overcome them: because greater is He that is in you, than he that is in the world."

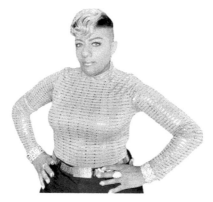

Dawn Thomas

HER2+ Breast Cancer

Be Encouraged ~
It's Going to be
Alright!

As I write this to encourage you, I am encouraging myself. My mother's firstborn, my oldest sister (she doesn't like when I say, "she's my oldest sister" (she prefers "sister"), is at her first "treatment" for ovarian cancer. I broke out in tears...of belief, of joy, of hope, and confidence: 1) because she looks so confident -I see it in her eyes. and 2) because I know in my heart of hearts, in the very epitome of my soul that she is going to be alright- and so will you.

This is a "process" in life that she and you are going through at this very moment in time, or you are in the "process of thriving - still, you are not giving up but are encouraged that you are going to be all right.

Four years ago, I, too, went through the "process." I, too, am thriving. The doctor called to let me know they found cancer, two types, and that I needed to see a team of specialists so that they could decide what type of treatment was right for me. I hung up the phone, sat in my car, looked up, and conversed with my Healer, the One who gave His life for me and you, asking for direction.

Decree: Jesus is the author and finisher of my faith, and by His stripes, I am healed.

I chose to have a bilateral mastectomy and hormone therapy so whatever your choice of treatment, your caregiver role, or your thriving journey, be encouraged and know it's going to be alright!

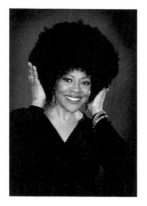

Dionne Shaw Bush

Conquer of breast cancer

Inspiring others with my faith, my strength, and my determination to live.

Facing The Giant

Lord, I thank you for teaching me that I must face the giant to be victorious. No matter how huge and intimidating this giant of cancer appears, You, Lord, have equipped me to fight and to win. As this giant stands in the fullness of who it is, I must also stand in the fullness of who I am in You; I will not back down, and I will not quit, for greater is He that is in me than He that is in the world. I must stand on Your promises that I am more than a conqueror through you, Lord, and though I am afraid, I will fight!

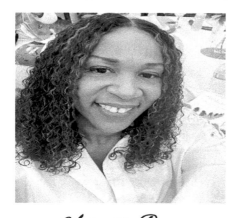

Antonitte Boone

2-time Breast Cancer Survivor, (2008)
Bilateral Mastectomy (2018)

Heaven Sent Champions

Living life as everyone else would

Striving to evolve as God said I should

Then came the most unexpected

Lord knows I did not want to accept it

You have cancer, a mass in your breast

We will call your doctor for the next steps

How could this be?

There is no biopsy, just a pic.

It's what we're trained to do,
no treat or trick.

Tears flooded my ears as
I lay on my back.

Devastated and shocked,
the doctor has no tact

The Father whispered
I'll take you through this

Oh God that means treatments, no omits

Anything that goes
through must come out

I had a solid promise of healing, no doubt

414 days of treatments,
chemo, and radiation

Days, I felt like one living in degradation

Suspended between Heaven and Earth

Coherent and clarity were dearth.

Yet God kept His promise
and kept my mind

I learned He was the reason
for daily Sonshine

My life never went back to the old norm

I just came through a horrific storm

The peace joy and power to live free

God showed the path of how to be me

The one He created for His glory

He knew I would tell the world
the beautiful story

To go on to a more perfected reflection

Of the Creator in this world of deception

Never stop the process
whatever it may be

God is the master strategist
to bring victory

For the man or woman
that will trust in Him

He brings out the fullest smile and grin

This causes Heaven and earth to rejoice

Everybody's gonna make some noise

Heaven sends champions just for the win

Stepping on sickness disease and chagrin

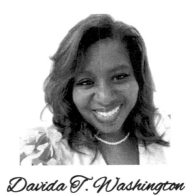

Davida T. Washington

Estrogen+ Breast Cancer Survivor January
29, 2023- 8 years

The Challenge

Life after breast cancer can be a challenge, but the fact that you're here is an infinite blessing. I ignored the signs for a while. My doctor gave me scripts, and I made excuses for why I didn't need them. I ignored the sharp pain in the middle of the night; I literally just turned over. God will bless you with angels in your ignorance, and that's what happened to me. A friend asked if I had surgery on my breast. My faith doesn't have words or dimensions, but it is all I need. The day I walked into my breast doctor's office, I was already prepared to fight.

I went through several chemotherapy sessions, surgery, and radiation. The most powerful day of my journey was when I shaved my hair. That was the day I felt most in control. The feeling of strength and liberation paved the way and gave me the strength to focus on living. I had too many people depending on me. I know my journeys are meant to prepare me to have the ability to share my light with many.

The first time I went back to see Dr. O., the shock of his face told it all. He said he honestly didn't know what he was going to do for me when he saw the size of the cancer. It literally covered the entire bottom of my breast. I said but doc, you told me I was stage two; he said I know what I told you. He gave me a hug and told me to keep doing what you are doing. It hasn't been easy, but it has been appreciated. Keep shooting for the star's pink sisters. The blessing, on the other side, is worth it. Keep sharing and caring.

I love you, and there is nothing you can do about it.

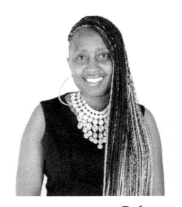

L. Charmaine Howard

Breast Cancer Survivor

Pink Is Still My Favorite Color!

I pray that my story will inspire, educate, empower, or comfort someone. It was a sunny day in the DMV on December 18th, and I had just returned home from emceeing the home-going of my dear friend and brother, Mr.

Edgar Brookins, aka Mr. DC from the AFRO American Newspaper, at the Fort Meyers Church. Unfortunately, he lost a long battle with prostate cancer. I was exhausted from standing and crying all day, so when I returned home, I asked my son, Chase, to please wake me up in two hours. I was supposed to meet my friends Roger Gore and Bahar Shaban at The Park at Fourteenth in Washington, DC; however, when my son woke me up, I felt a painful burning sensation from my belly bottom to my feet, and I could barely walk without feeling excruciating pain. I had no idea what was happening to me. I may have been experiencing a nightmare until I hit my hip on the bathroom sink and realized it was happening!

I called my girlfriend, Bahar, to let her know what was going on, and she told me not to call an ambulance and that she would be there shortly. She delivered me to the emergency room, where I would spend almost nine hours in the waiting area in excruciating pain. The incoming staff mistreated me. Two older white ladies were at the desk, and they treated me like I was faking to get to the front of the line. It was so humiliating to yelp in pain for so long and to be ignored as well as pointed at by other staff and patients. It was so horrible that I now refer to Shady Grove as Shady Grave. When the doctor finally was able to triage me and send me for X-rays, he was outraged that I had been sitting out in the waiting area while experiencing a fractured back in three places. Yes, my T8 has fractured in three places, and neither of us had a clue what happened to me. Once admitted, the customer service was still subpar, so I decided to research surrounding hospitals for back issues, equipment, etc., and leave and go to Holy Cross. Once I was finally checked in, my doctor hit the ground running, ordering tests, and processing my admission to the hospital, and I soon settled into a private room. Hallelujah! I was alone and could meditate and grasp what was happening without interruption.

I called my mom & sister Lisa (who lives with me) immediately to let them know what had occurred so they could disseminate the current information/status to the rest of the immediate family. Please understand that I didn't know much, but I wanted them to know I was settled in my room and in good spirits so they would not worry. It appeared out of nowhere, a medical team arrived at my door, and I was told that I would need to consider having surgery as soon as possible since my spinal cord was at risk of becoming severed. They only had to tell me that one time, and I was immediately scheduled for back surgery, which was Christmas Eve (December 24th, 2021). I was told it would be major back surgery. Before the surgery, I had to sign papers to acknowledge that I was aware of the possible complications, including becoming paralyzed. Wow! Ok, I signed the papers, began praying, and asked some of my tribe to pray. Several people visited me, which was indeed my saving grace that kept me sane because I think I was still in some twilight zone or shock!

Just minutes before I was prepared for surgery to go under the knife, I handed my surgeon a greeting card. What is so significant about this is that just before the anesthesia overwhelmed me, I saw that he had opened my card. It was placed on the counter of the operating room, and that made all the difference in calming my anxiety. Once I had this major back surgery, only a limited number of people knew, and several visited me, which lifted my spirits.

Thank you, my sister, Sonya, for bringing me food, balloons & flowers; Roger Gore, for your love & inspiration; my sister-friends Jeanna Robinson and Dr. Sylvia Traymore Morrison, for taking turns spending the night with me and Alexy Purohit, for spending time with me and giving me a hand and foot massage before the hospital stopped visitation privileges due to Covid. The only one who could visit was Rev. Dr. Rou because he had religious credentials.

My Medical Team was OUTSTANDING! Thank you to every doctor, nurse, aid, therapist, custodian, professional technician, administrative support staff, food handler & deliverer, transportation staff, and others. I especially would like to thank my surgeon, Dr. Jay Rhee, Washington, Brain & Spine Institute (and his amazing team), and my Primary medical physician, Dr. Surek Gupta (and his amazing team), who made my stay at Holy Cross as pleasant as possible. Holy Cross is an outstanding hospital with phenomenal staff!!!!!

After surgery, I could not walk! It was extremely difficult to move at all while in the hospital bed with my narcotic pump glued to my hand (lol). I found it difficult to become comfortable even with the many pillows the nurse gave me. That medicine pump became my Linus blanket in a Charlie Brown cartoon. Each week, I became stronger, received more care, such as physical and occupational therapy, and received a walker. I initially moved around like an inchworm, taking me what seemed like forever to maneuver my way to my hospital room door and back to the bed! My back was so painful 24/7 and felt heavy with the long strips of titanium fused to my spinal cord supporting my T8 to enable me to walk again. It's been almost two years (as of January 3, 2024), and I am still getting used to this foreign material in my body. I am grateful, though, because I could not walk without it. Thank you to the medical team & GOD!

On January 3rd, 2022, my doctor entered my room, and the "three words" he uttered would change my life as I knew it. He said, "You have cancer," and proceeded to explain what happened. The cancer was in my right breast and traveled through my lynch nodes and to my back (spine), whereas it fractured my T8 in three places. I proceeded to pick my mouth up from the floor and immediately started praying. Well, at least I knew what caused the break in my back, and now, I began asking the doctor a million questions and started a journal to record what was going on with me as much as possible.

Did I mention that I didn't have insurance? I lost my insurance after leaving my "good government job" in 2017 for a family emergency. I thank GOD for HIS Grace, Mercy, and Favor! My dear friend Rev. Dr. Bruce Branch located a contact so I could apply for Medicaid, and it was approved! It came right in the nick of time because the discharge employees kept coming into my room, harassing me to leave due to lack of insurance as if I was ready physically or even mentally to go. I was far from ready. Meanwhile, I was scheduled to have a port placed in my upper chest in preparation for when I started chemo and a slew of tests, x-rays, etc.

When I was finally ready to leave Holy Cross Hospital, it was my mother and sister, Lisa, who drove from Connecticut and were prepared to stay and nurse me back to health. They took me to my sister Sonya's home, where I would have lots of room to use my walker and could stay/sleep on her main floor since I could not use the stairs without experiencing pain. My sister Sonya was traveling quite a bit at the time with her job, so she allowed me to convalesce at her home. A nurse visited me twice during the first week to check my back and take vital signs. My Mom and my sister Lisa took me to my outpatient appointments; Lisa accompanied me to my first chemo treatment & dived my prescribed medication into a pill box; Mom cooked for me & and all three gave me encouragement and unconditional love every day.

They cared for my son and traveled back & forth to our condo to ensure that Chase was ok. I don't see how I would have managed or made it through without my family. #SupportisImportant #ButGOD A support system is a critical part of recovery. Also, PRAYER was, and will always be, everything for me! My mindset is stuck on the positive, and I focused on recovering 100%. I was at my sister Sonya's house for approximately three weeks, and on February 1st, 2022 (on my late Dad's birthday), I could walk without the walker. However, my doctor recommended that I continue to use it for at least ten additional days. #PraiseGOD I remember my second Great-nephew, Leo, was born the next day (February 2nd). That brought me so much JOY!

It was time for Mom and Lisa to return home to Connecticut and for me to return home to my condo with my son! I felt so bad when they returned to Connecticut and shared that pipes had burst in Lisa's home. They put their lives on hold for a month for me. They were helpful; Lisa set up my appointments and separated my medication into a medicine case. My Mom My Mom My Mom My Mom.... I cannot say her name enough!

There is NOTHING like a Mother's Love!

I received transportation to and from my weekly radiology appointments, my follow-up doctor's appointments, and, of course, chemo. It was a lonely and peculiar time to reflect, become disciplined with my diet, and change my routine. I experienced plenty of pivoting!

I was referred to my first holistic doctor by my longtime best friend, Marcella Barnes, and I decided to take a trip to California to meet Dr. Juan Perez and my new great-nephew, Leo. It was an awakening to hear an entirely different take on this illness. I was so grateful to learn so much positive information. It changed my whole perspective about my situation! I also recommend that everyone go to a holistic doctor to learn about holistic healing. It has been a tremendous asset in my life. Since leaving California, I have been determined to make the best of this situation and thrive! My family was most helpful throughout this journey. I want to thank them officially! Thank you to my mom (Ms. Charlotte Fraser aka Queen Bee), who has always put her family first, my sisters Lisa and Sonya, my nieces Amber (husband, Brandon & great-nephew Landon), Arielle (great-nephew Leo) and Shayna (husband Tray), & my son and heartbeat, Chase!

Shortly after my return home, I started feeling much stronger. I attended an event for the first time since my diagnosis was given to my dear sister, friend, Delegate & Assistant Speaker Pro Temp, Diana Fennell. Somehow, I mentioned my trip to California and the purpose, and to my surprise, she shared with me in confidence that she was experiencing the same illness. She graciously took me under her wing and introduced me to Dr. Kevin Streete, who has been a living angel in many ways to us and others. I attended a Governor-elect Wes Moore & Lt Governor Aruna Miller event in Oxon Hill. I was introduced to Patricia Plummer, and she, in turn, introduced me to Barbara Samaroo, who was another holistic covering. They were both fantastic, and Dr. Samaroo introduced me to a raindrop treatment and some natural treatments. I remember feeling horrible after a dose of chemo, so much so that I called Gayela Bynum, President of We Will Survive Cancer, to ask for Greg Babcock's contact info. He is a board member of We Will Survive

Cancer and was a huge help and wealth of knowledge as he survived cancer himself. He has quite a story in the first edition of the book Don't Waste Mt Cancer. He referred me to the Gentle Wellness Center; my experience was magical. They only accepted cash, so I was limited; however, after explaining their services and how they affect the body, I chose Vitamin C IV and Hyperbaric Oxygen therapy.

I couldn't believe how much better I felt afterward. Another precious gem was Dr. Angela Kalender, one of my sisters from Sisters 4 Sisters Network, Inc.

(S4SN). We became very close while traveling to Houston, Texas, to attend Dr. George C. Fraser's Power Networking Conference (PNC). She started to share priceless information with me regarding the illness and implemented physical treatment of a hand and foot massage during our stay in Houston, TX. Once all of us returned to Maryland (Peggy Morris, President S4SN; Sharon Bullock VP S4SN; Jeanie Bell-Waddell S4SN, Leris Bernard S4SN, Jackie Mims S4SN, Linda Powell S4SN, Connie Bell S4SN, Dr. Judith S4SN, Dr. Cheryl Wood S4SN, Dr. Chere Goode S4SN, Florence

Champagne S4SN and many more sisters), we met in person. I ordered holistic items to aid my health. She and her beautiful daughter performed a stomach regimen and oils with me that felt amazing! Thank you to Madam President Peggy Morris and the sisters (Sisters 4 Sisters Network, Inc.) for raising funds and the Christian Giving Circle to assist me with overdue bills. I have been blessed to have great friends support me in different ways; Thank you Dr. Remi Duyile, Stephanie White, Sonia Garbarino, Bershan Shaw, Karen Marie Alston, Dr. Renee Bovelle

(Ophthalmologist), Wayne Carter, Dawn Moss, LaKei ForestCosby, Rodney Burton, Ronald Byrd, Ozzy Ramos & AVB, Gina Rupert, Chef Selby, Josie Valdez, The #MooreMiller Campaign, raMona Designs (Celebrity Designer), Wendell & Elizabeth Carter, and so many many many more.

What can I say about Dr. Bruno Mazali? I call him Miracle Chef Mazali because he volunteered to cook healthy foods, smoothies, and nutritious juices for my son and me. and has been faithfully providing meals for many months. I believe he has been a huge part of my survival, and I am forever grateful. So many others have touched my life and continue to bless me! I thank them all! Please do not charge my heart if I did not mention you because I am grateful to everyone!

My son, Chase, became extremely helpful to me these past twenty-plus months since acclimating to our new life; both of us! My dear and longtime friend Dr. Lance London still calls me daily to check on me and give me words of encouragement; yes, every day! I also thank my friend Todd Rogers for his kindness and support. You know who your friends are when you become ill or in need!!!!!!! #MyGOD

How do I thank my sister-friends, Jackie Thompson & Dee Adams, for putting together a birthday fundraiser in 2022 to assist me with bills that became overdue since I couldn't work while hospitalized and unable to work for almost three months? Karen McConnell was instrumental in providing an interview on her radio show and secured letters from Judge Ingrid Turner, Dr. James Dula in the County Executives Veterans office and proclamations from Delegate Darryl Barnes, Peggy Morris

(President, S4SN) and States Attorney for Prince George's County, Aisha Braveboy to name a few. They raised funds, which I used to pay overdue bills. Everyone showered me with love, which gave me the boost I needed to start rebuilding!

Let's discuss the treatments, including radiation, chemo, and holistic elective procedures. My sister Lisa accompanied me to my first chemo treatment, and she was the perfect person to be with me because she followed my lead and was a tremendous & supportive gift to me. I felt calm when I met my assigned oncologist, Juneja, and it helped me get through that important day! I remember being quite anxious, knowing that I was about to allow poison into my body voluntarily. I kept thinking to myself that there must be a better way.... a cure after all this cancer research and all the billions of dollars poured into research and all. I entered the crowded room, and there was only one open chair for me. As I walked to that chair, passing other patients, it felt like dark clouds had parked themselves over the entire treatment room.

It felt as though most people in that room may have given up. It made me so sad! I took time that morning to put my make-up on my face and dress nicely to feel "good" despite what was about to occur. As the nurse connected the fluids to my IV, I started praying and then saying positive affirmations to myself. Then, I found myself praying for all the patients in the room and every person in the world who heard those three words; "You Have Cancer!" It has become a ritual part of chemo days (as Delegate Fennell calls SPA Day).

I know I've taken a lot of time to thank people, and I did that because it's critical to have a grateful heart while in this process. Without it, you could easily fall into a depression, have a pity party, and/or become an angry person. I know, as sure as my name is Renee, that I am alive because of my support and my mindset. Yes, the chemo, medicine, and holistic approach are essential, but my attitude has been the most critical ingredient in hindsight! I want everyone and anyone who has this illness or is caring for someone with this tumor (s) in their body to know that with a new diet, excellent care, and a new attitude, you can prolong your life. Bouncing back as soon as possible to a new normal to enjoy your life despite this is important!

One of the downfalls that I have found while maintaining my new normal and attempting to "just live my life" is that some people will question if you have the illness if you seem to be enjoying yourself too much! I have found this disturbing, a sign of jealousy and evilness. It's as though some people would rather see you balled up in a fetal position and distraught than to see you thriving. Go figure!

This past summer, two lesions were found on my brain, and on July 18th, 2023, I had radiation surgery to remove them. I want to thank the entire staff of Radiology Oncology: Nurse Jolice, Dr. Greer, Dr.

Moulds, Greg, Maia, Evelyn, Alba, Z, and the many angels on the dynamic team!

Please continue to fight through negativity or nonsense and do your best to ignore anyone who is not inspiring, encouraging, uplifting, educating, or positively assisting you. This includes your family, friends, oncologist, or otherwise. Fortunately, I have experienced much better than bad.

If any doctor or medical staff makes you feel less than others, please seek alternative care, but do so by referral. Dr. Street was vital to my comfort zone in choosing an additional doctor because I trusted him and am very pleased. There is nothing wrong with seeking a second opinion. Doctors are human; remember that! #PraiseGOD

To the family and friends of your loved ones with this illness, I ask that you provide unconditional love and remain open and flexible to their needs. It's an emotional roller-coaster for us to live with this every day. Some cry, laugh, etc... but whatever we do, we are learning to LIVE with this and recover! #InJusesName I often mask my feelings, so people won't feel sorry for me or start treating me differently. I can't speak for all people with this illness, but I can share that I want to live as normally as possible while helping others who are dealing with cancer or the aftermath of it as much as I can. I want to take this time to congratulate all the survivors and thrivers, honor our fallen angels, and send prayers to their families. GOD bless you, Kimberly Bennett, for all you have been through, and my deepest condolences to my friend Keula Binelly, who recently lost her husband, Scott. Too many people are suffering and losing their lives to this monster daily! Stay ENCOURAGED and FIGHT FOR YOUR LIFE through whatever means works for you!

I want to dedicate my chapter to all who are going through this illness in any way, as well as to my late Father, Mr. Leith Douglas Aloysius Fraser, who battled throat cancer like a champ before returning home in November 2016. I love you, Daddy, and miss you so much. You touched so many lives and continued philanthropic work in the community. You were my first love & hero! Rest in heavenly peace.

I recommend getting your paperwork in order if you hadn't before your diagnosis (your will, living will, trust, insurance, etc.). This has given me peace of mind because I no longer worry about it. I also suggest that you make a short-term and long-term list of things you want to do and/or complete in your lifetime. Some people call it a bucket list!

Lastly, I want to share that I have never (and shall never) lost my faith, and I credit that inner peace within me by possessing a strong belief in GOD! I pray that you have faith and cling to it like the oxygen you breathe because no one will if you don't believe in your healing. You must pull through this realistically with discipline, love, amazing new habits, and maybe even a new hobby! YOU CAN DO THIS! I thank GOD every day, sometimes several times, for His grace and Mercy. Favor isn't fair, and I am grateful for not looking like what I am going through! You can, too!

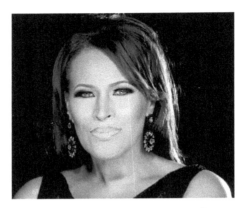

Dr. Renee' Starlynn Allen

President, Global Conscious Initiative

The Peoples Emcee in the DMV

Kingdom Ambassador White House Prayer
for our Nation

Radio & TV Host

Retired Veteran

Advocate for
Global Health & Human Decency

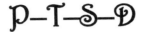

P–T–S–D

PERSEVERE

To continue a course of action in the face of difficulty and limited success.

Battling breast cancer is the most difficult obstacle I have ENCOUNTERED.

When support wavered, my commitment and willpower to WIN escalated.

Like "*The Little Engine That Could©*," I convinced myself...

"I KNOW I CAN – I KNOW I CAN, **PERSEVERE** and DEFEAT Breast Cancer!"

THRIVE

To prosper, flourish, and grow vigorously.

I'm making every attempt to maintain normalcy in my life. I created and fulfilled BUCKET LIST items ranging from eating exotic foods to traveling. To **THRIVE,** I must live in a constant state of joy and appreciation.

SURVIVE

To continue to live and exist despite danger or hardships.

In this journey called life, survival is the ULTIMATE GOAL. Prior to my breast cancer diagnosis, I was a survivor! I suffered strokes, paralysis, craniotomy surgeries, bilateral hip replacements, cardiac events, etc. Including my breast cancer illness, I have endured over 30+ surgical procedures. My mindset is always in survival mode – there is no other option.

I am a **SURVIVOR**! Thank GOD, I don't look like what I have been through.

DAILY

To complete/produce something that occurs every day.

YOU must PRAY – PRAY – and PRAY some more. My **DAILY** affirmation:

"For with GOD, ALL THINGS are POSSIBLE." Matthew 19:26, KJV

In order to **PERSEVERE, THRIVE,** and **SURVIVE** on a **DAILY** basis (P–T–S–D),

YOU must remind yourself, "I **HAVE CANCER – IT DOES NOT HAVE ME.**"

STAY ENCOURAGED. BE YOUR OWN ADVOCATE. LIVE in the MOMENT – YOU'VE GOT THIS!

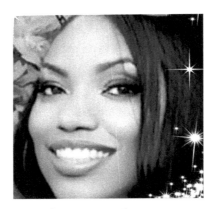

Patrice Antoinette

Breast Cancer Survivor 20 Years

Stage 2, Ductal Carcinoma in Situ Breast
Cancer (2003), Inflammatory Breast Cancer
(2005),

Bilateral Mastectomy (2013), Stage 4
Metastatic Breast Cancer (2016),

No Evidence of Active Disease
(NED) (May 2023)

Cancer of the Heart

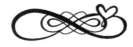

I've navigated through various challenges in my life, but THAT storm was unlike anything I'd faced. In those initial months, all I could muster was, "God, please help me." Prayer felt foreign, and my faith waned. My cancer journey was so overwhelming that bitterness and anger seeped in, directed at God and others. I clung to the hope of a miraculous intervention, believing that I might be a chosen recipient of God's rescuing grace, bypassing the conventional path to surviving cancer. It encompassed eleven relentless months of enduring excruciating chemotherapy, breast surgery, and unyielding radiation. Yet, as fate would have it, God had a different avenue of healing in store for me. I struggled to accept the abrupt disruption of my life's course.

Despite the bitterness, a flicker of love remained, compelling me to continue to attend church. It was during one of those services that I distinctly heard "cancer of the heart." This divine message hit me so hard, and through my tears, it dawned on me that I must extend an invitation to the ultimate Healer, welcoming Him back into the depths of my heart. I embraced His offer, surrendering my bitterness, resentment, anger, embarrassment, and fears. In return, He bestowed upon me true, genuine healing and restoration. This wasn't just about physical recovery; God wanted to uproot the anger and bitterness at the core of my being. While I yearned for a swift physical recovery, God aimed to address the deeper emotional wounds hindering complete healing.

Indeed, healing encompasses both time and the chances we seize. Often, it feels simpler to succumb to negativity rather than embrace positivity through struggle. This journey, dear sister, was sanctioned by God. His profound love is exhibited in His concern for our self-presentation before Him. For what He truly desires is our heart.

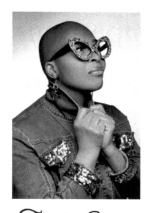

Teresha Sutton

9-year Breast Cancer Thriver

Companionship
Versus Isolation

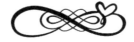

Keep in mind your breast cancer journey affects not only you but your family and friends. Allow and trust your family and friends to be on your team just like you allow and trust your medical team with your life.

Embrace and welcome the love and support from your family and friends. The initial diagnosis and prognosis of your breast cancer journey do lead you to the behavior of seclusion. It is imperative not to remain in that state. Recognizing that you are worthy and deserving of being loved is essential. Being the recipient of different acts of love and surrounding yourself with family and close friends will enhance your healing process. Realize that you are one of the most special people in the world to your family and close friends. Embrace and encompass your entire being with the special blessings loved ones bestowed upon you. Remember, "The Lord is good to all, and his tender mercies are over all his works. Psalm 145.9. "And He will love thee and bless thee. **Deuteronomy 7:13**.

On 3-6-2006, I decided to isolate myself and my illness from family and friends once I received my diagnosis. Weeks later, I realized that isolation was not my best decision. Through a lot of soul-searching and spiritual guidance, I chose companionship. In retrospect, I learned how to embrace the aspects of companionship and how it progressed my healing process in a strong spiritual manner. Currently, I am living my best life currently as a 17-year breast cancer survivor.

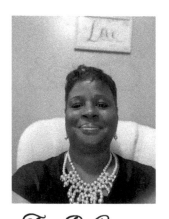

Tina D. Carter

17 Years in Remission

STAGE 2 Breast Cancer

Words of Encouragement

CANCER... When I heard that six-letter word, I fell to the floor, got on my knees, and cried God's word of healing. I knew I was not finished living a full life. God is not finished with YOU! I am a survivor. You will survive, too.

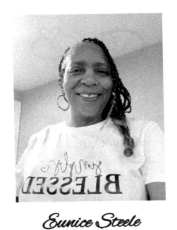

Eunice Steele

Breast Cancer Survivor

Survivor

The mere fact you're reading this is because you are a SURVIVOR!

God gives his hardest battles to his strongest soldiers. You've survived 100% of everything that has been thrown at you. Every day, rise with prayer, praise, and gratitude. You are a warrior. Just remember this: you're never alone! I pinky promise you that! I'm my sister's keeper for life.

Quote: "The human spirit is stronger than anything that happens to it. "-Author C.C Smith

BE BLESSED YOU GOT THIS. I will be cheering you on the whole way!

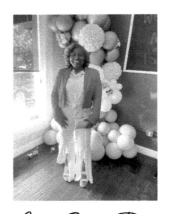

Lakey Green Poole

Breast Cancer Thriver

Know That It Is OK

You are probably dealing with an array of emotions right now if you have been recently diagnosed or are starting the treatment process for breast cancer. I know that I dealt with shock, anxiety, disbelief, disappointment, embarrassment, guilt, and fear to name a few.

Know that it is OK to feel what you feel.

Know that you can get through this.

Know that you are not alone.

Then, make a decision to OVERCOME and WIN.

Make a decision to be a VICTOR, not a VICTIM.

Here are 21 actions that helped me get through my 12 rounds of Chemo/Immunotherapy treatment in 2023.

1. Let your FAITH be bigger than your FEAR.

2. Identify your support system and keep them close to you and in the loop.

3. Accept that your body will go through many changes.

4. Follow your Doctor's and Infusion Nurse's orders/instructions.

5. Find out what vitamins and supplements are safe to take during your treatment. Vitamin D was a lifesaver for me.

6. Ask questions about what to expect from each medicine and treatment.

7. Make going to your infusions a "FUN ACTIVITY." Take a family member or friend with you for a conversation. Plan an after-treatment activity.

8. Use your infusion time to do something you've been putting off, like reading a book, writing, making phone calls, organizing paperwork, doing arts and crafts, etc.

9. Reward yourself after each infusion treatment.

10. Journal your side effects after each infusion. It will help you see

patterns in your response to the medicines.

11. Drink lots of WATER and EAT throughout your treatment weeks. Not only will it help you stay hydrated, but it will also "feed your soul."

12. Keep fresh melon fruit, ginger, and soursop tea in your home.

13. REST when you're tired.

14. If you are working, consider taking an Intermittent Leave of Absence to call out as needed without being penalized.

15. GET UP and GO when you can. Walking, sunlight, and light exercise or stretching are good for your body.

16. Elevate your feet as much as possible to prevent excessive swelling in your ankles.

17. GET CUTE & COMFY for your infusions. When you look better, you feel better.

18. Wake up each day with a purpose or goal. It will push you to get through this.

19. Celebrate your successes along the way.

20. **KNOW THAT THIS IS JUST 1 YEAR OF YOUR ENTIRE LIFE** and that this treatment will give you a new lease on life.
21. Ask God daily for COMPLETE HEALING, RESTORATION, **and RENEWAL**.

"Life is about accepting your reality and making the necessary adjustments.

The ones who navigate the best will get the best out of life".

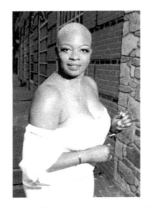

Shauna "Getchalifeon" Starks

Breast Cancer Thriver

The Journey

The breast cancer journey can be rewarding yet overwhelming. My journey began in 2012 when I became aware that I had breast cancer. When I was first diagnosed, I was terrified of the unknown. HELL, I had breast cancer! I asked myself, "WHAT DO I DO NOW?" After I found out that I had this dreaded disease, my chemo began. I can recall during my first round of chemo, and I was also in the process of trying to launch my newly found business, SOLES 4 DIVAS, which included launching my website and securing inventory and vendors for various events. Simply put, I was trying to do everything required to start a business. While doing multiple things for the business, I began to get sick from the chemo treatments. Again, another "WHAT DO I DO NOW MOMENT" Imagine trying to launch a shoe business while being treated for cancer.

After realizing that I had cancer, along with a family to take care of- GIVING UP WAS NOT AN OPTION. I couldn't give up for a few reasons: 1) I realized that GOD hadn't brought me this far to leave me, 2) I wanted to finish implementing the gifts that GOD had granted me, and 3) I had children who depended on me. Having gone through this, my faith kicked into overdrive, and I needed to get my business off the ground. I continued to work on the business. I finalized my website and ensured I had inventory for the various events I was scheduled to participate in. While working on the business, believe it or not, no one knew that I had breast cancer. Yes, I kept this a secret from the outside world. I didn't want folks to have "pity" on me. While having cancer, I officially launched SOLES4 DIVAS in May 2012. YES - I launched a full business with having breast cancer, BUT GOD. The business's launch was highly successful; I offered unique footwear for DIVAS worldwide. Sales were insane, and I was happy. I honestly couldn't keep up with the demands of my customers. I had no idea that SOLES4 DIVAS would be on fire so soon. This made me excited despite having cancer. Honestly, the launch of my business gave me hope; it also provided an outlet that caused me not to think about having cancer, as well as bringing in extra income for my household. The year 2012 was a solid rollercoaster, from being diagnosed with breast cancer to launching an international online shoe boutique. I was looking forward to all the possibilities that 2013 would bring.

2013 was a new year with a new beginning. I was excited! The business was still thriving, and my cancer, although having become a vital part of my being (at this point), I didn't allow having cancer to stop me. I knew that I needed to continue. At this point, I not only had my family who depended on me, but My business needed me, as well. Talk about balance. September 13, 2013, was when my dreams transitioned into reality. I BECAME A BREAST CANCER SURVIVOR! I no longer had to go to chemo treatments or hospital appointments (which included being poked with a million needles, etc.). And the ultimate, the relief of the financial burden from expensive medication that I had to take. Talk about being relieved. (THANK YOU, JESUS). I no longer had to encounter any of this—a **BIG** sigh of relief.

What Now...

The business was still thriving; having gone through everything that I went through, GOD allowed the business to thrive. At this point, I no longer needed public assistance. I was relieved that I no longer had to "wait" for the government to give me what I needed. Although I worked my butt off up until this point in my life, I needed that help during that time. I was now finally able to maintain my monthly expenses on my own. Talk about a shift. The change that was occurring physically, mentally, spiritually, and financially was exhilarating.

Who is Damitra?

Thinking back to that point, I can now stand firmly and say that GOD allowed me to weather the storm. I AM A BREAST CANCER SURVIVOR and Chief Executive Officer (C.E.O) of SOLES 4 DIVAS, LLC. Founder and Visionary Officer of Soles 4 The Cure, which is a non-profit that provides support systems to assist women of color with breast cancer. Talk about leveling up in business. Since its launch, SOLES 4 DIVAS, LLC., has been featured in the international New York Fashion Week for five consecutive years, has added styling as a service offered to customers for red carpet and various events, and continues hosting fashion shows domestically and internationally. As a breast cancer survivor, it is important to share my story with those individuals who have been affected by cancer and teach them to live life beyond the diagnosis. When not running my business, I enjoy spending time with my family and friends, who have been instrumental during my journey. This is a REAL example of combining your PASSION and

PURPOSE to make your business PROFITABLE (the triple "P" effect.). My story also shows you that you can overcome obstacles, have faith, trust the process, and allow GOD to do the rest.

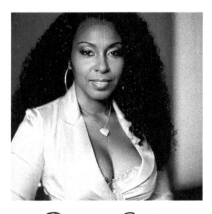

Damitra Sorden

The Sole Survivor

God Will
Bless You

I am a richly blessed breast cancer survivor, and this year (April 2023) marks my 25-year breast cancer survivor anniversary.

My abundance of faith and amazingly supportive family and friends have been the driving force to keep me strong and claim victory over this life-threatening disease.

Each day, I am so thankful to embrace the quality of life with my beautiful family, and I praise God for giving me the tenacity to live my life to the fullest.

Throughout the highs and lows of my journey, it was therapeutic to engage in positive activities to manage my spirit of healing.

When the challenges soared my life out of the ordinary, the keyword that helped me prevail was temporary. (i.e., mastectomy, hair loss, weight loss, skin discoloration) – All that was lost was later regained or restored.

I praise God (the master Surgeon) for His healing hands and am most grateful for my phenomenal, caring, and comforting healthcare medical team.

My passion is to uplift awareness, raise funds, and advocate for those affected by breast cancer.

Let breast cancer not be the darkness of life interference, but put on your armor of faith and hope and be the warrior of perseverance.

As we continue the fight to beat breast cancer, let's empower those affected by this disease to instill, inspire, endure, and walk with faith to find a cure".

Know your vision and self-worth in everything you do and walk in your purpose, and God will continue to Bless you.

Blessing of Love,

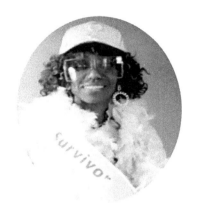

Diane Wallace

25-Year Breast Cancer Survivor

Healed and
Restored

To God Be the Glory for the great things he has done. I was living my best life while pursuing a degree as a Psychiatric Nurse Practitioner with an online program at Wilkes University. My life was interrupted by a diagnosis of left breast cancer in September 2022. I can honestly say that God has been with me during this journey. A porta catheter was placed in my right chest for chemotherapy. I received my first dose of chemotherapy on Wednesday, 9-7-2022, and proceeded to Pennsylvania on 9-11-2022 to receive my certification as a Psychiatric Nurse Practitioner. I can remember my grandchildren asking about my chest surgical dressing. I gave a smile and said that God is helping me to fight breast cancer. I completed IV chemotherapy, radiation treatment, and a lumpectomy in less than six months. God has empowered me to withstand this journey. The Joy of the Lord has been my strength. I managed to continue to work and maintain all the bills with the help of my husband. I am presently on a course of chemotherapy by mouth to ensure that the cancer remains in remission. I can say with confidence that God is Faithful. The scripture that I am standing on is:

Isaiah 53:5

But He was wounded for my transgressions; He was bruised for my iniquities; The chastisement for my peace was upon him, and I am healed and restored by his stripes.

Thank you, Jesus!

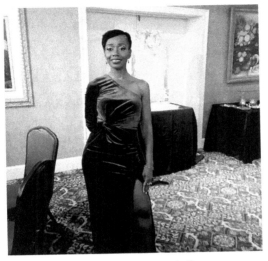

Starlene McKelvin

Breast Cancer Survivor

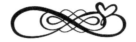

Dear Readers,

I am overwhelmed with gratitude as I reflect on the incredible journey we've embarked on together through the pages of "Pinky Promises." Your support, encouragement, and willingness to embrace the message of empowerment and sisterhood have touched my heart in ways I cannot express.

As the Women's Wellness Lounge founder and the visionary behind the She Is Well book project, I am continually inspired by the strength and resilience of women like you who dare to dream big and strive for a life of wellness and fulfillment.

Thank you for allowing me to be a part of your lives and entrusting me with your stories, struggles, and triumphs. I hope that "Pinky Promise" has served as a source of inspiration, encouragement, and empowerment as you navigate the twists and turns of your wellness journey.

As we continue to uplift and support one another, may we always remember the strength and resilience within each of us. Together, we can overcome any obstacle and achieve our dreams, one pinky promise at a time.

With deepest gratitude,

Delayna Watkins

Founder, Women's Wellness Lounge
Visionary, She Is Well Book Project
www.womenswellnesslounge.org

PLEDGE

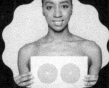

I PINKY PROMISE TO:

EMBRACE MY BREAST HEALTH IN THE FOLLOWING WAYS

 LEARN RISKS AND FAMILY HISTORY

 PERFORM MONTHLY BREAST SELF EXAMS

 ANNUAL CLINICAL EXAMS TO INCLUDE MAMMOGRAMS

 ADOPT A HEALTHY LIFESTYLE

 TAKE OFF MY BRA AND BECOME FAMILIAR WITH MY BREASTS

**LEARN MORE ABOUT THE PINKY PROMISE PROJECT:
WWW.WOMENSWELLNESSLOUNGE.ORG**

Printed in the USA
CPSIA information can be obtained
at www.ICGtesting.com
CBHW051109081124
17082CB00020B/421